Nature's Cure: Herbal Remedies for Piles and Hemorrhoids

GLORIA DAVIES

Introduction

The Prevalence and Impact of Piles or Hemorrhoids on Daily Life

Piles, also known as hemorrhoids, are a common condition affecting millions of people worldwide. These swollen veins in the lower rectum and anus can cause significant discomfort, pain, and bleeding.

For many, the simple act of walking or sitting becomes a challenge, and using the restroom can be an ordeal filled with fear and anxiety. The constant discomfort and inconvenience can severely impact one's quality of life, making everyday activities seem difficult.

Introduction to Natural Healing Methods and Their Benefits

In the quest for relief, many turn to conventional treatments like ointment cream, drug medications, or even surgery. While these methods can be effective, they often come with side effects and do not address the underlying causes.

This is where natural healing methods shine. Utilizing herbs and other natural ingredients offers a holistic approach to treating piles. These methods are gentle on the body, often with fewer side effects, and they work to improve overall health rather than just masking symptoms.

Overview of the Book and Natural Remedies for Piles/Hemorrhoids

In this book, we'll explore a variety of natural remedies specifically tailored for the treatment of piles and hemorrhoids.

You'll learn about powerful herbs like bitter kola and red onions, which have been used for generations to provide relief.

We'll delve into the science behind these remedies, how to prepare them, and the best ways to incorporate them into your daily routine.

Additionally, we'll cover lifestyle and dietary changes that can help prevent the recurrence of piles, providing a comprehensive guide to maintaining digestive health. This book aims to empower you with knowledge and practical solutions, so you can take control of your health and find lasting relief from the discomfort of piles.

By the end of this journey, you'll have natural remedies to help you live more comfortably and healthily, free from the pain and inconvenience of hemorrhoids or piles.

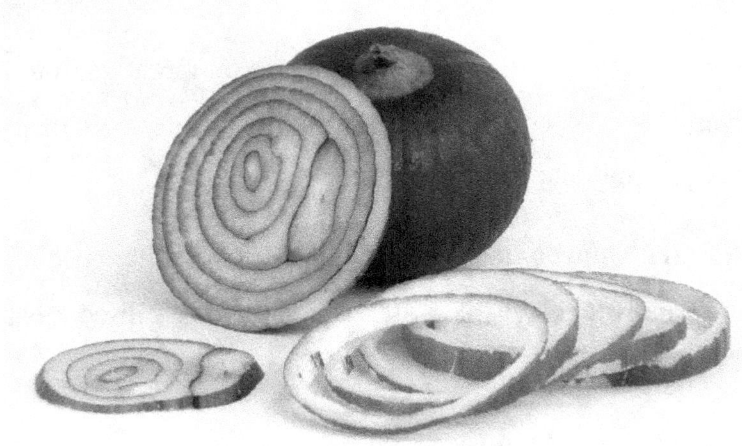

CHAPTER 1

Understanding Piles/Hemorrhoids

Definition and Types of Hemorrhoids

Hemorrhoids, commonly referred to as piles, are swollen and inflamed veins located around the anus or in the lower rectum.

They are similar to varicose veins that you might see on a person's legs. Hemorrhoids are classified into two main types: internal and external.

Internal Hemorrhoids: These are located inside the rectum. They usually aren't visible or felt and rarely cause discomfort unless they are prolapsed or severe.

External Hemorrhoids: These form under the skin around the anus and can be quite painful, itchy, and uncomfortable.

Common Causes

Several factors contribute to the development of hemorrhoids. Some of the most and common causes include:

Diet: A low-fiber diet can lead to constipation, which can cause straining during bowel movements, increasing the pressure on the veins in the rectum and anus.

Lifestyle: Sedentary lifestyles or prolonged sitting can increase the risk. Lack of physical activity can also contribute to constipation.

Genetics: Some people inherit a possible tendency to develop hemorrhoids.

Pregnancy: The increased pressure on the pelvic blood vessels during pregnancy can cause hemorrhoids.

Aging: Hemorrhoids are more common in older adults because the tissues supporting the veins in the rectum and anus can weaken with age.

Symptoms and Stages of Hemorrhoids

Hemorrhoids can present a variety of symptoms, and their severity can range from mild discomfort to significant pain and inconvenience.

Symptoms:

- Bleeding during bowel movements.
- Itching or irritation in the anal region.
- Pain or discomfort.
- Swelling around the anus.
- A lump near the anus may appear, which may be sensitive or painful.

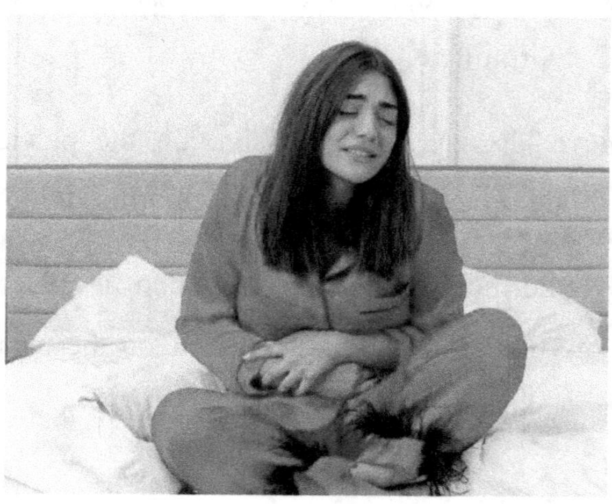

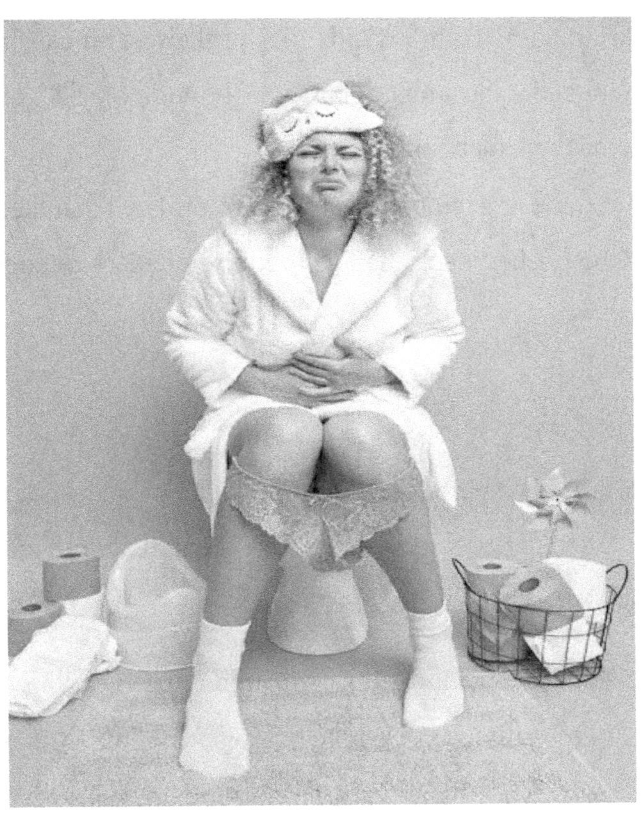

Stages:

- Grade 1: Small inflammations inside the lining of the anus that are not visible.

- Grade 2: Larger than grade 1 but still inside the anus. They may get pushed out during bowel movements but return on their own.

- Grade 3: Hemorrhoids that prolapse and can be felt outside the anus. They can be temporarily pushed back in manually.
- Grade 4: Hemorrhoids that are prolapsed and cannot be pushed back in. They require medical treatment.

Complications if Left Untreated

If hemorrhoids are not treated properly, they can lead to more serious health problems. Some potential complications include:

- Chronic Blood Loss: Continuous bleeding from hemorrhoids can lead to anemia, a condition in which you don't have enough red blood cells to carry oxygen throughout your body.
- Strangulated Hemorrhoid: If the blood supply to an internal hemorrhoid is cut off, it can cause extreme pain and lead to tissue death.
- Infection: Both internal and external hemorrhoids can become infected, which can lead to further complications such as abscesses.

- Prolapse: Severe cases of internal hemorrhoids can prolapse, or extend beyond the anus, which may require surgical intervention.

Understanding these aspects of hemorrhoids can help in recognizing the condition early and seeking appropriate treatment to prevent complications. The next sections will delve into natural remedies and lifestyle changes that can help manage and alleviate the symptoms of piles.

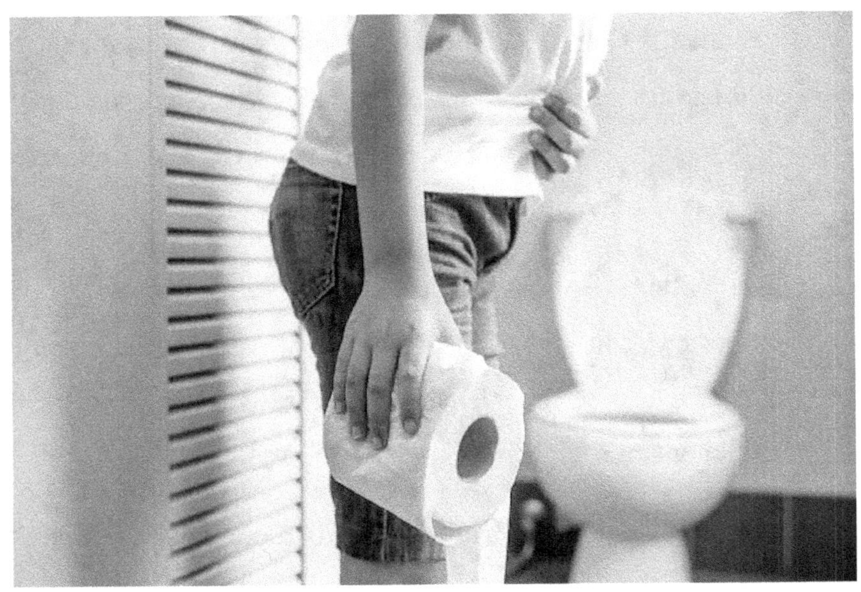

CHAPTER 3

Conventional Treatments

Overview of Common Medical Treatments

When it comes to treating hemorrhoids, there are several conventional medical options available. These range from over-the-counter remedies to surgical procedures, depending on the severity and persistence of the condition.

Creams and Ointments: These are usually the first line of treatment for hemorrhoids. Products containing hydrocortisone or witch hazel can help reduce inflammation and soothe irritation. Hemorrhoid creams often provide temporary relief from pain and itching.

Medications: A pain reliever like acetaminophen or ibuprofen can help manage pain. Additionally, stool softeners or fiber supplements can ease bowel movements, reducing strain on hemorrhoids.

Minimally Invasive Procedures: For more persistent cases, doctors may recommend procedures such as rubber band ligation, where a small band is placed around the base of a hemorrhoid to cut off its blood supply.

Sclerotherapy, which involves injecting a solution into the hemorrhoid to shrink it, and infrared coagulation, which uses heat to cause hemorrhoids to retract, are also common.

Surgery: In severe cases, surgical procedures like hemorrhoidectomy (removal of hemorrhoids) or stapled hemorrhoidopexy (stapling hemorrhoids back into place) might be necessary. These are generally considered when other treatments have failed or when hemorrhoids are particularly large and painful.

Limitations and Side Effects of Conventional Treatments

While conventional treatments can be effective, they often come with limitations and potential side effects such as:

- Temporary Relief: Many creams and ointments provide only short-term relief, addressing symptoms rather than the underlying issue.

- Side Effects: Prolonged use of topical steroids like hydrocortisone can lead to skin thinning. Pain medications can cause gastrointestinal issues, and stool softeners may lead to dependency.

- Invasive Procedures: Minimally invasive treatments can be uncomfortable and sometimes require multiple sessions. Surgical options, while effective, carry risks such as infection, pain, and prolonged recovery time.

Cost and Accessibility: Some treatments, particularly surgical options, can be expensive and may not be accessible to everyone.

Why Natural Remedies Are a Viable Alternative

Natural remedies offer a holistic approach to treat hemorrhoids, addressing both the symptoms and underlying causes without many of the downsides associated with conventional treatments.

Fewer Side Effects: Herbal treatments and dietary changes typically come with fewer side effects compared to pharmaceuticals and invasive procedures.

Cost-Effective: Natural remedies often involve readily available ingredients and lifestyle adjustments, making them more affordable.

Holistic Health Benefits: By focusing on overall digestive health, natural remedies can provide long-term relief and prevent recurrence. For example, increasing fiber intake not only helps with hemorrhoids but also improves overall bowel health.

Empowerment: Learning about and using natural remedies can empower individuals to take control of their health through diet, lifestyle changes, and the use of beneficial herbs.

In this book, we will explore various natural remedies, such as the use of bitter kola and red onions, which have been traditionally used to treat hemorrhoids effectively. We'll also delve into dietary and lifestyle changes that can help manage and prevent hemorrhoids, offering a comprehensive and sustainable approach to health.

CHAPTER 4

The Power of Natural Remedies

Benefits of Using Herbs and Natural Ingredients

When it comes to managing and treating hemorrhoids, natural remedies offer several advantages.

Herbs and natural ingredients can provide effective relief while being gentle on the body.

These treatments often come with fewer side effects compared to conventional medications. They work holistically, promoting overall health rather than just addressing specific symptoms.

Additionally, natural remedies are often more affordable and accessible, making them a practical choice for many people.

Historical and Cultural Significance of Herbal Remedies

Herbal remedies have been used for centuries across various cultures for their healing properties. Traditional medicine systems, such as Ayurveda in India and Traditional Chinese Medicine, have long relied on herbs to treat a range of ailments, including hemorrhoids.

These practices are rooted in the belief that natural ingredients can restore balance to the body and promote healing from within.

The use of herbs is also prevalent in African, Native American, and many other indigenous medical traditions. This rich history underscores the enduring trust in and effectiveness of herbal remedies.

Introduction to the Key Ingredients: Bitter Kola and Red Onions

In our exploration of natural treatments for hemorrhoids, two key ingredients stand out: bitter kola and red onions.

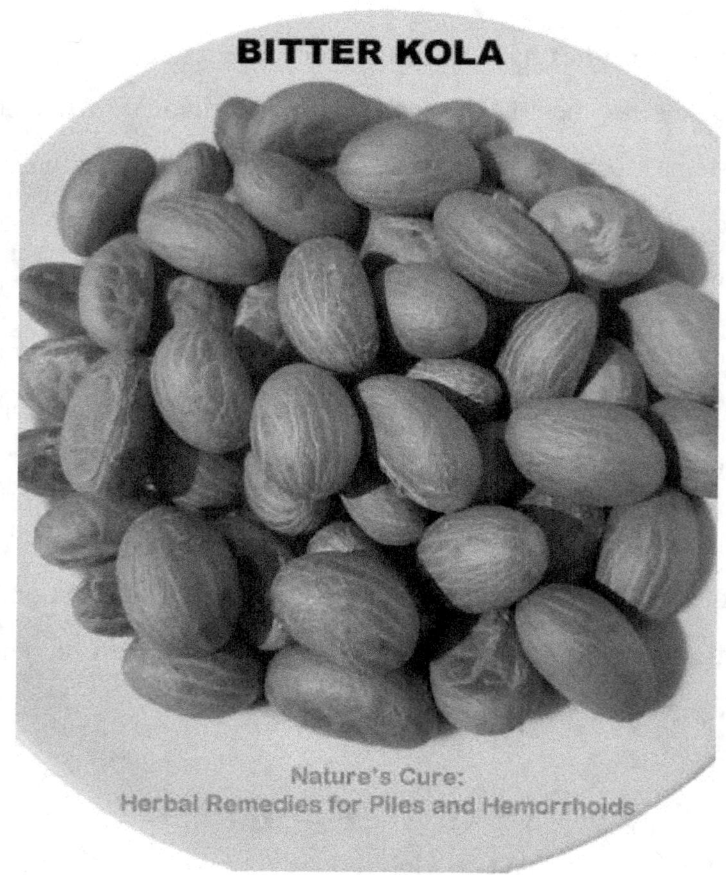

Bitter Kola: Also known as Garcinia kola, bitter kola is a plant commonly found in West Africa. It has been used for centuries for its medicinal benefits and properties.

Bitter kola is known for its anti-inflammatory and antioxidant benefits, which can help reduce the swelling and discomfort associated with hemorrhoids. It is also believed to improve circulation, which can aid in the healing process.

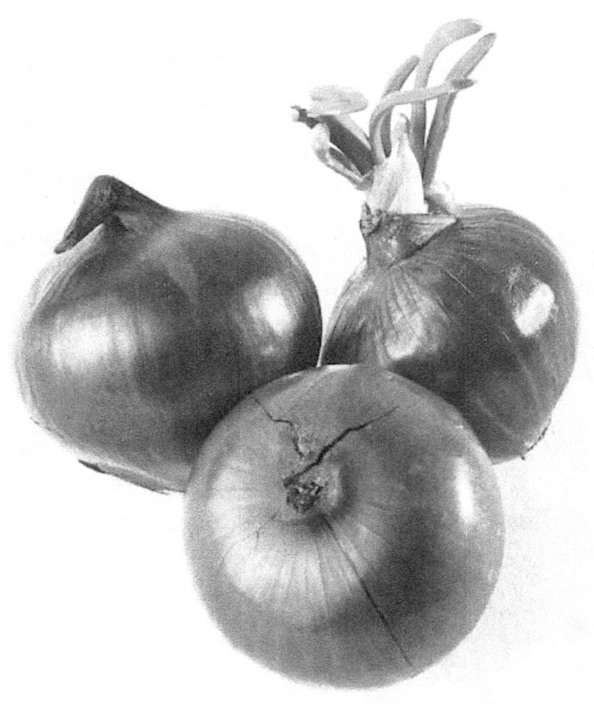

RED ONION

Red Onions: Red onions are not only a culinary staple but also a powerful natural remedy.

They are rich in quercetin, a flavonoid with strong anti-inflammatory properties. Consuming red onions can help reduce inflammation and soothe irritated tissues.

They also have antimicrobial properties, which can help prevent infections that might complicate hemorrhoids.

In this book, we will delve deeper into how these natural ingredients can be used to treat hemorrhoids effectively. We will provide practical recipes and guidelines for incorporating them into your daily routine, helping you take a natural and holistic approach to health and wellness.

CHAPTER 5

Bitter Kola: Nature's Healer

Botanical Description and Origins of Bitter Kola

Bitter kola, scientifically which known as Garcinia kola, is a flowering plant native to West and Central Africa. It grows as a medium-sized tree, reaching up to 30 meters in height. The plant produces small, round fruits that encase the bitter-tasting seeds for which the tree is named. These seeds, commonly referred to as bitter kola nuts, have a distinctive bitter flavor and have been valued for their medicinal properties for centuries.

Nutritional and Medicinal Properties

Bitter kola is packed with nutrients and active compounds that contribute to its medicinal benefits. It contains high levels of vitamins A, C, and E, which are essential for maintaining good health. Additionally, it is rich in antioxidants, which help protect the body from oxidative stress and free radicals.

The nuts also contain significant amounts of potassium, calcium, and caffeine, making them a natural stimulant.

Medicinally, bitter kola is renowned for its anti-inflammatory, antimicrobial, and antiviral properties. These attributes make it effective in treating a range of ailments, from infections to inflammatory conditions. It is also known to improve digestion, boost the immune system, and support respiratory health.

Traditional Uses of Bitter Kola in Various Cultures

Throughout Africa, bitter kola has been an integral part of traditional medicine for generations. In Nigeria, it is commonly used to treat chest colds and coughs.

Healers also use it to combat digestive issues and as a general health tonic. In Ghana, the seeds are chewed to relieve the symptoms of asthma and bronchitis.

Beyond its medicinal uses, bitter kola holds cultural significance. It is often used in social and spiritual ceremonies, symbolizing hospitality and respect.

Offering bitter kola to guests is a traditional gesture of goodwill and friendship in many West African communities.

Scientific Studies Supporting Its Effectiveness

Modern scientific research has begun to validate the traditional uses of bitter kola. Studies have shown that the seeds possess potent anti-inflammatory and antimicrobial properties.

Research published in the Journal of Ethnopharmacology demonstrated that bitter kola extract could inhibit the growth of certain bacteria and fungi, supporting its use in treating infections.

Another study in the African Journal of Biochemistry Research highlighted the antioxidant properties of bitter kola, which can help in reducing oxidative stress and preventing chronic diseases.

Additionally, a clinical trial published in the Nigerian Journal of Clinical Practice found that bitter kola effectively improved symptoms in patients with osteoarthritis, thanks to its anti-inflammatory effects.

In summary, bitter kola is a powerful natural remedy with a rich history of use in traditional medicine. Its nutritional and medicinal properties are well-documented, and scientific research continues to support its effectiveness in treating a variety of health conditions. This makes bitter kola an invaluable tool in natural healing practices.

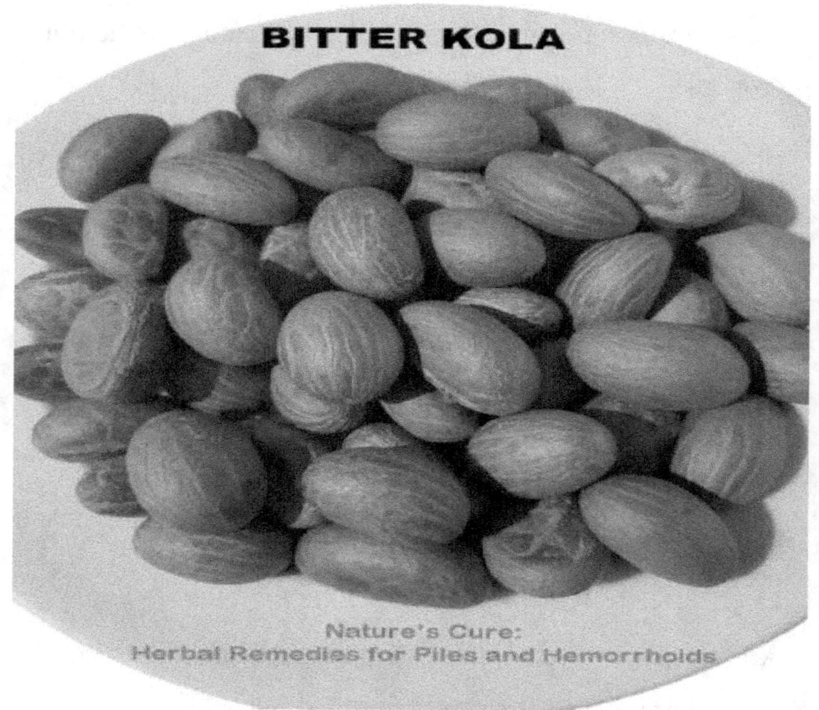

CHAPTER 6

Nutritional Profile and Health Benefits of Red Onions

Red onions are more than just a colorful addition to your salad; they are packed with nutrients that offer numerous health benefits.

These vibrant vegetables are rich in vitamins C and B6, as well as folate and potassium. They also provide a good amount of dietary fiber, which is essential for maintaining healthy digestion. Moreover, red onions are low in calories, making them a nutritious choice for any diet.

Medicinal Properties and Traditional Uses

Historically, red onions have been used in various traditional medicine practices around the world. Their medicinal properties have made them a staple in home remedies for centuries.

The high levels of quercetin, a potent antioxidant and anti-inflammatory compound found in red onions, contribute to their health benefits. Quercetin helps reduce inflammation and may lower the risk of chronic diseases such as heart disease and cancer.

In traditional medicine, red onions have been used to treat a variety of ailments. They are often utilized to alleviate symptoms of respiratory conditions such as colds and asthma. The antimicrobial properties of red onions make them effective in fighting infections. Additionally, they have been used to promote wound healing and improve overall immune function.

How Red Onions Aid in Reducing Inflammation and Improving Digestion

Red onions are particularly beneficial for reducing inflammation and improving digestion, two key factors in managing and preventing hemorrhoids.

Reducing Inflammation: The quercetin in red onions acts as a natural anti-inflammatory agent. It helps to reduce swelling and irritation in the body, including in the veins affected by hemorrhoids. By incorporating red onions into your diet, you can help mitigate the inflammation that contributes to the discomfort of hemorrhoids.

Improving Digestion: Red onions are rich in dietary fiber, which is crucial for maintaining healthy digestion. Fiber adds bulk to the stool and promotes regular bowel movements, reducing the strain during defecation that can exacerbate hemorrhoids.

Additionally, the prebiotic fibers in red onions feed beneficial gut bacteria, which play a vital role in digestive health.

By including red onions in your diet, you can harness their natural healing properties to support overall health and alleviate the symptoms of hemorrhoids.

Whether eaten raw in salads, cooked in meals, or even used as a natural remedy, red onions provide a powerful, herbal ally in the journey towards better health.

CHAPTER 7

Preparation and Usage Guide

Detailed Step-by-Step Guide to Preparing the Remedy

Ingredients:

- 3 bitter kola nuts
- 3 red onions
- Clean water

Preparation:

Grinding the Bitter Kola:

Start by thoroughly washing the bitter kola nuts to remove any dirt or impurities.

Use a grinder or mortar and pestle to grind the bitter kola nuts into a fine powder.

Ensure that the powder is consistent and free of large chunks.

Slicing the Red Onions:

Peel the red onions and wash them well.

Slice the onions into small, even pieces. This helps in releasing their beneficial compounds during boiling.

Boiling Instructions:

Place the ground bitter kola and sliced red onions into a pot.

Add clean water, not more than 3 liters, to the pot.

Boil the both bitter kola and red onion for at least 30 minutes. This allows the beneficial compounds from the bitter kola and red onions to infuse into the water.

After 30 minutes, remove the pot from the heat and let the mixture cool very well or slightly.

Dosage:

Drink one teacup of the prepared remedy twice a day. This dosage ensures that you receive the benefits of the remedy without overwhelming your system.

Safety Precautions and Tips for Usage

Start Slowly: If you are new to using natural remedies, start with a smaller dose to ensure that your body tolerates it well.

Monitor Your Reaction: Please pay attention to your body and how your body responds to the remedy. If you experience any strange or adverse reactions, discontinue drinking it and consult a healthcare professional immediately.

Stay Hydrated: Drink plenty of water throughout the day to help your body flush out toxins and stay hydrated.

Storage and Shelf Life of the Prepared Remedy

Storage: Store the prepared remedy in a clean, airtight container to maintain its potency. Please keep it in the refrigerator to preserve it for a long time use.

Shelf Life: The remedy can be stored for up to one week in the refrigerator. Discard any unused portion after this period and prepare a fresh batch if needed.

By following this guide, you can effectively prepare and use a natural remedy that harnesses the healing properties of bitter kola and red onions. This approach provides a holistic and accessible way to manage the symptoms of hemorrhoids and support overall digestive health.

CHAPTER 8

Additional Herbal Remedies and Practices

Other Beneficial Herbs for Piles

Witch Hazel: Witch hazel is a popular natural remedy for hemorrhoids due to its astringent properties, which help to reduce swelling and inflammation. Applying witch hazel extract topically can provide relief from pain and itching.

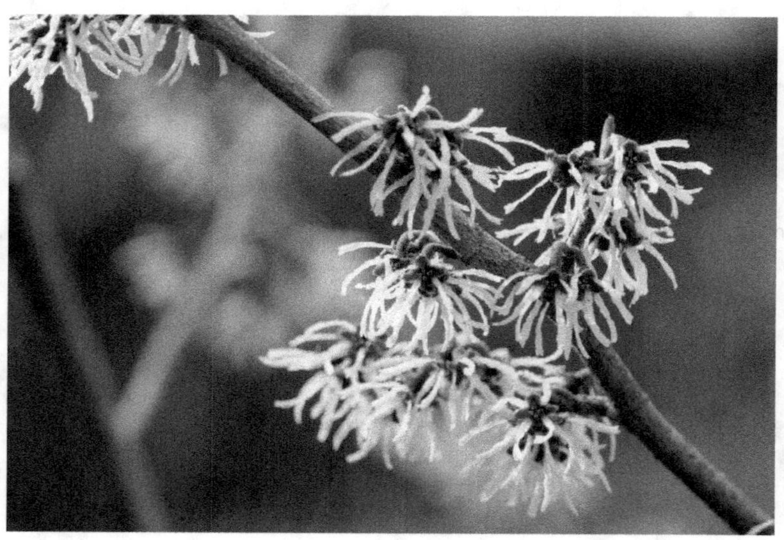

WITCH HAZEL IMAGE

Horse Chestnut: This herb is known for its ability to strengthen blood vessels and improve circulation. Horse chestnut extract can reduce swelling and discomfort associated with hemorrhoids.

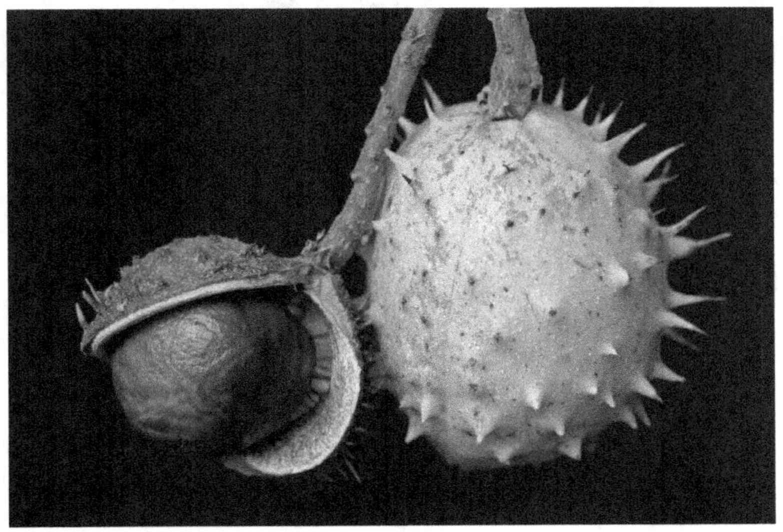

Horse Chestnut Image

Butcher's Broom: Butcher's broom has anti-inflammatory and vasoconstrictive properties, making it effective in reducing the symptoms of hemorrhoids. It can be taken as a supplement or used in topical preparations.

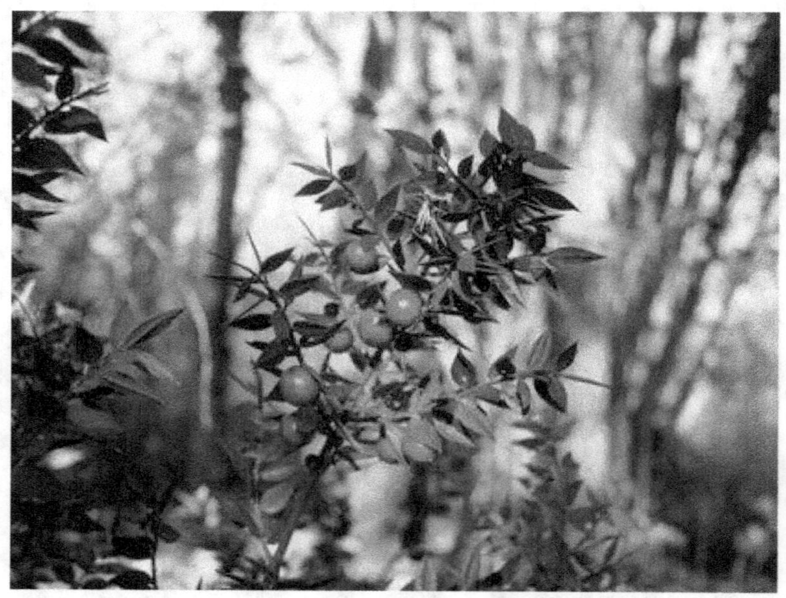

Butcher's Broom Image

Combining Herbs for Enhanced Effectiveness

Using a combination of these herbs can enhance their overall effectiveness.

For example, a topical ointment containing witch hazel and butcher's broom can provide both immediate relief and long-term healing benefits.

Similarly, combining horse chestnut with dietary changes can improve blood vessel health and reduce the likelihood of hemorrhoid flare-ups.

DIY Herbal Ointments and Topical Applications

Making your own herbal ointments can be a cost-effective way to manage hemorrhoids. Here's a simple recipe:

Ingredients:

- 1 tablespoon of witch hazel extract
- 1 tablespoon of butcher's broom extract
- 1 tablespoon of coconut oil (optional, for soothing application)

Instructions:

- Mix the witch hazel and butcher's broom extracts in a small bowl.
- Add the coconut oil if you prefer a soothing base.
- Apply the mixture to the affected area using a clean cotton pad.

Dietary Recommendations for Supporting Digestive Health

Maintaining a healthy diet is crucial for preventing and managing hemorrhoids. Here are some dietary tips:

High-Fiber Foods: Include plenty of fruits, vegetables, whole grains, and legumes in your diet to ensure regular bowel movements and reduce straining.

Hydration: Drink a lot of water throughout the day to keep your stools soft and prevent constipation.

Avoid Irritants: Reduce your intake of spicy foods, caffeine, and alcohol, as these can irritate the digestive system and exacerbate hemorrhoid symptoms.

Lifestyle Changes to Prevent Recurrence

Hydration: Staying well-hydrated helps maintain healthy digestion and prevents constipation, a major cause of hemorrhoids.

Exercise: Regular physical activity can improve circulation and digestive health. Target at least 30 minutes of moderate exercise in at least 3 or 4 days a week.

Stress Management: Chronic stress can negatively impact digestive health. Practice more of stress-reducing techniques such as meditation, yoga, or deep breathing exercises.

Proper Bathroom Habits: Avoid straining during bowel movements and try not to sit on the toilet for extended periods. Consider using a footstool to elevate your feet and create a more natural squatting position.

By incorporating these additional herbal remedies and lifestyle practices into your routine, you can effectively manage and prevent hemorrhoids, promoting overall digestive health and well-being.

CHAPTER 9

Case Studies and Success Stories

Real-Life Testimonials from Individuals Who Have Benefited from the Remedy

Jane's Journey to Healing:

Ms. Jane, a 45-year-old teacher, had been struggling with severe hemorrhoids for years. She had tried various over-the-counter treatments and even considered surgery.

Upon learning about the natural remedy involving bitter kola and red onions, she decided to give it a try. Within a few weeks, Jane experienced significant relief.

Her symptoms of pain and swelling decreased, and she was able to return to her daily activities without discomfort.

Jane credits the natural remedy for giving her a new lease on life and helping her avoid invasive procedures.

Michael's Relief Story:

Michael, a young professional, often suffered from hemorrhoid flare-ups due to his sedentary lifestyle and poor diet. After incorporating the herbal remedy into his routine, Michael noticed an improvement in his digestive health and a reduction in hemorrhoid symptoms.

The combination of dietary changes, increased fiber intake, and the use of the natural remedy helped Michael manage his condition effectively. He now advocates for natural treatments and encourages others to explore holistic approaches.

Stories from Farming Communities and Their Traditional Practices

Wisdom of the Elders:

In many farming communities across West Africa, traditional knowledge about natural remedies has been passed down through generations.

One such community shared their experience with using bitter kola and red onions to treat hemorrhoids.

The elders explained that this remedy has been a staple in their healthcare practices for decades. They prepare the mixture as a regular part of their diet, not just as a treatment but also as a preventive measure.

The community's collective health has benefited from these practices, with fewer cases of severe hemorrhoids and other digestive issues.

A Village Healer's Testimony:

A respected healer from a rural village recounted numerous success stories of individuals who had come to him for help with hemorrhoids.

Using the traditional bitter kola and red onion remedy, he had treated hundreds of patients.

The healer shared how the natural ingredients, combined with a healthy lifestyle, brought relief to many. His testimony underscores the importance of traditional practices and their relevance even in modern times.

Encouraging Narratives to Inspire Readers

Emma's Empowering Experience:

Emma, a mother of two, felt helpless when conventional treatments failed to alleviate her hemorrhoid symptoms. Frustrated and in pain, she turned to natural remedies as a last resort.

The results were astonishing. Not only did the bitter kola and red onion remedy provide relief, but it also empowered Emma to take control of her health.

She began to educate herself about natural treatments and made holistic health a priority for her entire family.

Emma's story is a testament to the power of natural remedies and the positive impact they can have on one's life.

A Community's Transformation:

In a small town where hemorrhoids were a common issue due to dietary habits, a local health initiative introduced the natural remedy of bitter kola and red onions.

The community embraced this approach, incorporating the remedy into their daily routines. Over time, there was a noticeable decline in hemorrhoid cases and an overall improvement in digestive health.

This success story highlights the potential for community-wide transformation through the adoption of natural health practices.

These case studies and success stories illustrate the effectiveness of natural remedies in treating hemorrhoids.

They offer hope and inspiration, showing that with the right knowledge and approach, it is possible to find relief and improve quality of life naturally.

CHAPTER 10

Precautions and When to Seek Medical Help

Understanding the Limitations of Herbal Remedies

While herbal remedies can be highly effective for many people, it's important to understand their limitations. Natural treatments often work best for mild to moderate cases and as part of a holistic approach to health.

They can take longer to show results compared to conventional medicines, and the effectiveness can vary from person to person.

Moreover, herbal remedies may not address the root cause of a severe condition and might not be sufficient for advanced cases of hemorrhoids.

Recognizing Signs That Require Professional Medical Attention

It's crucial to know when to seek professional medical help for hemorrhoids. The following signs indicate a need for medical attention:

Persistent Pain and Bleeding: If you experience severe or prolonged pain, or if there is significant bleeding during bowel movements, it's important to consult a healthcare professional.

Changes in Bowel Habits: Sudden changes in bowel habits, such as persistent diarrhea or constipation, can indicate an underlying condition that requires medical evaluation.

Prolapsed Hemorrhoids: If the hemorrhoids protrude from the anal opening and do not retract, this could require surgical treatment.

Infection: Signs of infection, such as increased pain, swelling, redness, or fever, necessitate immediate medical attention.

Ignoring these symptoms can lead to complications, such as anemia from chronic blood loss or thrombosed hemorrhoids, which are painful blood clots within the hemorrhoid.

Integrating Herbal Treatments with Conventional Medicine Safely

Combining herbal treatments with conventional medicine can provide a balanced approach to managing hemorrhoids. Here are some tips for safe integration:

Consult Your Doctor: Before starting any herbal remedy, discuss it with your healthcare provider, especially if you are already on medication or have other health conditions.

Some herbs can interact with medications and affect their efficacy or cause adverse effects.

Follow Dosage Guidelines: Stick to recommended dosages for both herbal remedies and medications to avoid overuse or potential toxicity.

Monitor Your Health: Keep track of any changes in your symptoms or overall health. If you notice any adverse reactions, stop the herbal remedy and consult your doctor.

Use High-Quality Products: Ensure that the herbs and natural products you use are of high quality and sourced from reputable suppliers to avoid contamination or substandard ingredients.

By understanding the role and limitations of herbal remedies, recognizing when to seek medical help, and safely integrating natural treatments with conventional medicine, you can effectively manage hemorrhoids and support your overall health.

CHAPTER 11

Resources and Further Reading

Reliable Sources for Purchasing Bitter Kola and Red Onions

Finding high-quality bitter kola and red onions is crucial for the effectiveness of natural remedies. Here are some reliable sources:

Local Health Food Stores: Many health food stores carry bitter kola and organic red onions. These stores often source their products from reputable suppliers.

Online Retailers: Websites like Amazon, Etsy, and specialized herbal shops offer bitter kola and organic red onions. Always check customer reviews and ratings to ensure quality.

Farmers' Markets: Local farmers' markets are excellent places to find fresh, organic red onions. Some markets may also have vendors selling bitter kola.

Recommended Books, Websites, and Research Articles on Herbal Medicine

For those interested in delving deeper into the world of herbal medicine, the following resources can be very informative:

Books:

"Herbal Medicine: Biomolecular and Clinical Aspects" by Iris F. F. Benzie and Sissi Wachtel-Galor – This book provides a comprehensive overview of the science behind herbal medicine.

"The Complete Herbal Tutor" by Anne McIntyre – A practical guide to using herbs for health and wellness.

"The Herbal Apothecary" by JJ Pursell – A detailed guide to medicinal herbs and their uses.

Websites:

National Center for Complementary and Integrative Health (NCCIH): NCCIH offers evidence-based information on various herbs and natural treatments.

HerbMed: HerbMed is an interactive, electronic herbal database that provides access to scientific data on the use of herbs for health.

Research Articles:

PubMed: PubMed is a free search engine accessing primarily the MEDLINE database of references and abstracts on life sciences and biomedical topics, including herbal medicine studies.

Journal of Ethnopharmacology: This journal publishes articles on the traditional use of medicinal plants and other substances.

Professional Organizations and Support Groups for Individuals with Hemorrhoids

Joining professional organizations and support groups can provide additional information and emotional support for individuals dealing with hemorrhoids:

Professional Organizations:

American Gastroenterological Association (AGA): AGA offers resources and information on gastrointestinal health, including hemorrhoids.

American Society of Colon and Rectal Surgeons (ASCRS): ASCRS provides information on surgical and non-surgical treatments for hemorrhoids.

Support Groups:

Hemorrhoids Support Group on Facebook: This online community provides a platform for individuals to share experiences, advice, and support.

Reddit's Hemorrhoids Community: Reddit has a community where individuals discuss treatments, symptoms, and support related to hemorrhoids.

By utilizing these resources, readers can further educate themselves on natural remedies, connect with supportive communities, and find high-quality ingredients to manage and treat hemorrhoids effectively.

CHAPTER 12

Conclusion

Recap of the Natural Approach to Treating Piles

Throughout this book, we've explored a range of natural remedies and holistic practices designed to alleviate and manage hemorrhoids.

From the healing properties of bitter kola and red onions to the benefits of incorporating high-fiber foods and maintaining a healthy lifestyle, these natural approaches offer effective, sustainable solutions for a condition that affects many.

By addressing both the symptoms and underlying causes, these methods promote overall digestive health and provide lasting relief without the harsh side effects often associated with conventional treatments.

Encouragement to Embrace Holistic Health Practices

Embracing holistic health practices can transform not only how you manage hemorrhoids but also your overall well-being.

The power of natural remedies lies in their ability to work with your body's natural processes, fostering long-term health improvements.

By integrating these practices into your daily routine, you can experience enhanced vitality, improved digestive health, and a greater sense of control over your health journey.

Final Thoughts and Words of Encouragement

Taking the first step towards natural healing can be daunting, especially if you've been relying on conventional treatments for years.

However, as you've seen through the case studies and success stories, many have found significant relief and improved quality of life by turning to nature's remedies.

Remember, healing is a journey, and every small step towards better health is a victory.

Take control of your health by empowering yourself with information and knowledge.

Trust in the process, and be patient with yourself as you incorporate these natural remedies and lifestyle changes.

You have the tools and information needed to manage and prevent hemorrhoids naturally.

Embrace this opportunity to take control of your health, and look forward to a future free from the discomfort and pain of hemorrhoids.

Wishing you health, healing, and happiness on your journey to better well-being.

CHAPTER 13

Journal for Managing Piles/Hemorrhoids with Natural Remedies

Day 1: Getting Started

Date:

Mood:

Why I'm Starting This Journey:

- What prompted you to try natural remedies for hemorrhoids?

....

....

....

....

....

....

....

Baseline Symptoms:

- Current pain level (1-10):
- Frequency and severity of bleeding: [Yes/No]
- Itching or discomfort: [Yes/No]
- Bowel movement difficulties: [Yes/No]

Reflection: Today marks the beginning of my journey with natural remedies to treat hemorrhoids. I'm hopeful that this approach will provide relief and improve my overall health. My main goals are to reduce pain and discomfort, and prevent future occurrences.

Day 2: First Day of Natural Treatment

Date: [Enter Date]

Mood: [Enter Mood]

Herbal Remedy Used:

Ingredients:

- Bitter Kola
- Red Onions
- Water

Preparation:

- Ground the bitter kola
- Sliced the onions
- Boiled them together

Dosage:

- Drank one tea cup in the morning and one in the evening

Observations:

- Did you feel any different before taking the remedy? [Yes/No]
- Did you feel any different after taking the remedy? [Yes/No]
- Any immediate changes or effects? [Yes/No]

Day 3: Daily Check-In

Date: [Enter Date]:

Mood: [Enter Mood]:

Symptom Update:

- Pain level (1-10): [Enter Number]
- Changes in bleeding: [Yes/No]
- Changes in discomfort: [Yes/No]
- Easier bowel movements: [Yes/No]

Diet and Lifestyle Changes:

- High-fiber foods added to diet: [Yes/No]
- Hydration habits improved: [Yes/No]
- Regular exercise: [Yes/No]

Reflection:

....

....

....

....

....

....

Day 4: Daily Check-In

Date: [Enter Date]:

Mood: [Enter Mood]:

Symptom Update:

- Pain level (1-10): [Enter Number]
- Changes in bleeding: [Yes/No]
- Changes in discomfort: [Yes/No]
- Easier bowel movements: [Yes/No]

Diet and Lifestyle Changes:

- High-fiber foods added to diet: [Yes/No]
- Hydration habits improved: [Yes/No]
- Regular exercise: [Yes/No]

Reflection:

....

....

....

....

....

....

Day 5: Daily Check-In

Date: [Enter Date]:

Mood: [Enter Mood]:

Symptom Update:

- Pain level (1-10): [Enter Number]
- Changes in bleeding: [Yes/No]
- Changes in discomfort: [Yes/No]
- Easier bowel movements: [Yes/No]

Diet and Lifestyle Changes:

- High-fiber foods added to diet: [Yes/No]
- Hydration habits improved: [Yes/No]
- Regular exercise: [Yes/No]

Reflection:

....

....

....

....

....

....

Day 6: Daily Check-In

Date: [Enter Date]:

Mood: [Enter Mood]:

Symptom Update:

- Pain level (1-10): [Enter Number]
- Changes in bleeding: [Yes/No]
- Changes in discomfort: [Yes/No]
- Easier bowel movements: [Yes/No]

Diet and Lifestyle Changes:

- High-fiber foods added to diet: [Yes/No]
- Hydration habits improved: [Yes/No]
- Regular exercise: [Yes/No]

Reflection:

....

....

....

....

....

....

Day 7: Daily Check-In

Date: [Enter Date]:

Mood: [Enter Mood]:

Symptom Update:

- Pain level (1-10): [Enter Number]
- Changes in bleeding: [Yes/No]
- Changes in discomfort: [Yes/No]
- Easier bowel movements: [Yes/No]

Diet and Lifestyle Changes:

- High-fiber foods added to diet: [Yes/No]
- Hydration habits improved: [Yes/No]
- Regular exercise: [Yes/No]

Reflection:

....

....

....

....

....

....

Day 8: Daily Check-In

Date: [Enter Date]:

Mood: [Enter Mood]:

Symptom Update:

- Pain level (1-10): [Enter Number]
- Changes in bleeding: [Yes/No]
- Changes in discomfort: [Yes/No]
- Easier bowel movements: [Yes/No]

Diet and Lifestyle Changes:

- High-fiber foods added to diet: [Yes/No]
- Hydration habits improved: [Yes/No]
- Regular exercise: [Yes/No]

Reflection:

....

....

....

....

....

....

Day 10: Daily Check-In

Date: [Enter Date]:

Mood: [Enter Mood]:

Symptom Update:

- Pain level (1-10): [Enter Number]
- Changes in bleeding: [Yes/No]
- Changes in discomfort: [Yes/No]
- Easier bowel movements: [Yes/No]

Diet and Lifestyle Changes:

- High-fiber foods added to diet: [Yes/No]
- Hydration habits improved: [Yes/No]
- Regular exercise: [Yes/No]

Reflection:

....

....

....

....

....

....

Day 11: Daily Check-In

Date: [Enter Date]:

Mood: [Enter Mood]:

Symptom Update:

- Pain level (1-10): [Enter Number]
- Changes in bleeding: [Yes/No]
- Changes in discomfort: [Yes/No]
- Easier bowel movements: [Yes/No]

Diet and Lifestyle Changes:

- High-fiber foods added to diet: [Yes/No]
- Hydration habits improved: [Yes/No]
- Regular exercise: [Yes/No]

Reflection:

....

....

....

....

....

....

Day 11: Daily Check-In

Date: [Enter Date]:

Mood: [Enter Mood]:

Symptom Update:

- Pain level (1-10): [Enter Number]
- Changes in bleeding: [Yes/No]
- Changes in discomfort: [Yes/No]
- Easier bowel movements: [Yes/No]

Diet and Lifestyle Changes:

- High-fiber foods added to diet: [Yes/No]
- Hydration habits improved: [Yes/No]
- Regular exercise: [Yes/No]

Reflection:

....

....

....

....

....

....

Day 12: Daily Check-In

Date: [Enter Date]:

Mood: [Enter Mood]:

Symptom Update:

- Pain level (1-10): [Enter Number]
- Changes in bleeding: [Yes/No]
- Changes in discomfort: [Yes/No]
- Easier bowel movements: [Yes/No]

Diet and Lifestyle Changes:

- High-fiber foods added to diet: [Yes/No]
- Hydration habits improved: [Yes/No]
- Regular exercise: [Yes/No]

Reflection:

....

....

....

....

....

....

Day 13: Daily Check-In

Date: [Enter Date]:

Mood: [Enter Mood]:

Symptom Update:

- Pain level (1-10): [Enter Number]
- Changes in bleeding: [Yes/No]
- Changes in discomfort: [Yes/No]
- Easier bowel movements: [Yes/No]

Diet and Lifestyle Changes:

- High-fiber foods added to diet: [Yes/No]
- Hydration habits improved: [Yes/No]
- Regular exercise: [Yes/No]

Reflection:

....

....

....

....

....

....

Day 14: Daily Check-In

Date: [Enter Date]:

Mood: [Enter Mood]:

Symptom Update:

- Pain level (1-10): [Enter Number]
- Changes in bleeding: [Yes/No]
- Changes in discomfort: [Yes/No]
- Easier bowel movements: [Yes/No]

Diet and Lifestyle Changes:

- High-fiber foods added to diet: [Yes/No]
- Hydration habits improved: [Yes/No]
- Regular exercise: [Yes/No]

Reflection:

....

....

....

....

....

....

Day 15: Challenges and Adjustments

Date: [Enter Date]

Mood: [Enter Mood]

Difficulties Encountered:

- Struggles with maintaining the regimen: [Yes/No]
- Any adverse reactions or side effects: [Yes/No]

Adjustments Made:

- Changes to the remedy dosage or preparation: [Yes/No]
- Modifications to diet or exercise routine: [Yes/No]

Positive Changes Noted:

- Significant improvements in symptoms: [Yes/No]
- Positive feedback from others: [Yes/No]

Reflection:

....

....

....

....

....

Day 16: Daily Check-In

Date: [Enter Date]:

Mood: [Enter Mood]:

Symptom Update:

- Pain level (1-10): [Enter Number]
- Changes in bleeding: [Yes/No]
- Changes in discomfort: [Yes/No]
- Easier bowel movements: [Yes/No]

Diet and Lifestyle Changes:

- High-fiber foods added to diet: [Yes/No]
- Hydration habits improved: [Yes/No]
- Regular exercise: [Yes/No]

Reflection:

....

....

....

....

....

....

Day 17: Daily Check-In

Date: [Enter Date]:

Mood: [Enter Mood]:

Symptom Update:

- Pain level (1-10): [Enter Number]
- Changes in bleeding: [Yes/No]
- Changes in discomfort: [Yes/No]
- Easier bowel movements: [Yes/No]

Diet and Lifestyle Changes:

- High-fiber foods added to diet: [Yes/No]
- Hydration habits improved: [Yes/No]
- Regular exercise: [Yes/No]

Reflection:

....

....

....

....

....

....

Day 18: Daily Check-In

Date: [Enter Date]:

Mood: [Enter Mood]:

Symptom Update:

- Pain level (1-10): [Enter Number]
- Changes in bleeding: [Yes/No]
- Changes in discomfort: [Yes/No]
- Easier bowel movements: [Yes/No]

Diet and Lifestyle Changes:

- High-fiber foods added to diet: [Yes/No]
- Hydration habits improved: [Yes/No]
- Regular exercise: [Yes/No]

Reflection:

....

....

....

....

....

....

Day 19: Daily Check-In

Date: [Enter Date]:

Mood: [Enter Mood]:

Symptom Update:

- Pain level (1-10): [Enter Number]
- Changes in bleeding: [Yes/No]
- Changes in discomfort: [Yes/No]
- Easier bowel movements: [Yes/No]

Diet and Lifestyle Changes:

- High-fiber foods added to diet: [Yes/No]
- Hydration habits improved: [Yes/No]
- Regular exercise: [Yes/No]

Reflection:

....

....

....

....

....

....

Day 20: Daily Check-In

Date: [Enter Date]:

Mood: [Enter Mood]:

Symptom Update:

- Pain level (1-10): [Enter Number]
- Changes in bleeding: [Yes/No]
- Changes in discomfort: [Yes/No]
- Easier bowel movements: [Yes/No]

Diet and Lifestyle Changes:

- High-fiber foods added to diet: [Yes/No]
- Hydration habits improved: [Yes/No]
- Regular exercise: [Yes/No]

Reflection:

....

....

....

....

....

....

Day 21: Daily Check-In

Date: [Enter Date]:

Mood: [Enter Mood]:

Symptom Update:

- Pain level (1-10): [Enter Number]
- Changes in bleeding: [Yes/No]
- Changes in discomfort: [Yes/No]
- Easier bowel movements: [Yes/No]

Diet and Lifestyle Changes:

- High-fiber foods added to diet: [Yes/No]
- Hydration habits improved: [Yes/No]
- Regular exercise: [Yes/No]

Reflection:

....

....

....

....

....

....

Day 22: Daily Check-In

Date: [Enter Date]:

Mood: [Enter Mood]:

Symptom Update:

- Pain level (1-10): [Enter Number]
- Changes in bleeding: [Yes/No]
- Changes in discomfort: [Yes/No]
- Easier bowel movements: [Yes/No]

Diet and Lifestyle Changes:

- High-fiber foods added to diet: [Yes/No]
- Hydration habits improved: [Yes/No]
- Regular exercise: [Yes/No]

Reflection:

....

....

....

....

....

....

Day 23: Daily Check-In

Date: [Enter Date]:

Mood: [Enter Mood]:

Symptom Update:

- Pain level (1-10): [Enter Number]
- Changes in bleeding: [Yes/No]
- Changes in discomfort: [Yes/No]
- Easier bowel movements: [Yes/No]

Diet and Lifestyle Changes:

- High-fiber foods added to diet: [Yes/No]
- Hydration habits improved: [Yes/No]
- Regular exercise: [Yes/No]

Reflection:

....

....

....

....

....

....

Day 24: Daily Check-In

Date: [Enter Date]:

Mood: [Enter Mood]:

Symptom Update:

- Pain level (1-10): [Enter Number]
- Changes in bleeding: [Yes/No]
- Changes in discomfort: [Yes/No]
- Easier bowel movements: [Yes/No]

Diet and Lifestyle Changes:

- High-fiber foods added to diet: [Yes/No]
- Hydration habits improved: [Yes/No]
- Regular exercise: [Yes/No]

Reflection:

....

....

....

....

....

....

Day 25: Daily Check-In

Date: [Enter Date]:

Mood: [Enter Mood]:

Symptom Update:

- Pain level (1-10): [Enter Number]
- Changes in bleeding: [Yes/No]
- Changes in discomfort: [Yes/No]
- Easier bowel movements: [Yes/No]

Diet and Lifestyle Changes:

- High-fiber foods added to diet: [Yes/No]
- Hydration habits improved: [Yes/No]
- Regular exercise: [Yes/No]

Reflection:

....

....

....

....

....

....

Day 26: Daily Check-In

Date: [Enter Date]:

Mood: [Enter Mood]:

Symptom Update:

- Pain level (1-10): [Enter Number]
- Changes in bleeding: [Yes/No]
- Changes in discomfort: [Yes/No]
- Easier bowel movements: [Yes/No]

Diet and Lifestyle Changes:

- High-fiber foods added to diet: [Yes/No]
- Hydration habits improved: [Yes/No]
- Regular exercise: [Yes/No]

Reflection:

....

....

....

....

....

....

Day 27: Daily Check-In

Date: [Enter Date]:

Mood: [Enter Mood]:

Symptom Update:

- Pain level (1-10): [Enter Number]
- Changes in bleeding: [Yes/No]
- Changes in discomfort: [Yes/No]
- Easier bowel movements: [Yes/No]

Diet and Lifestyle Changes:

- High-fiber foods added to diet: [Yes/No]
- Hydration habits improved: [Yes/No]
- Regular exercise: [Yes/No]

Reflection:

....

....

....

....

....

....

Day 28: Daily Check-In

Date: [Enter Date]:

Mood: [Enter Mood]:

Symptom Update:

- Pain level (1-10): [Enter Number]
- Changes in bleeding: [Yes/No]
- Changes in discomfort: [Yes/No]
- Easier bowel movements: [Yes/No]

Diet and Lifestyle Changes:

- High-fiber foods added to diet: [Yes/No]
- Hydration habits improved: [Yes/No]
- Regular exercise: [Yes/No]

Reflection:

....

....

....

....

....

....

Day 29: Daily Check-In

Date: [Enter Date]:

Mood: [Enter Mood]:

Symptom Update:

- Pain level (1-10): [Enter Number]
- Changes in bleeding: [Yes/No]
- Changes in discomfort: [Yes/No]
- Easier bowel movements: [Yes/No]

Diet and Lifestyle Changes:

- High-fiber foods added to diet: [Yes/No]
- Hydration habits improved: [Yes/No]
- Regular exercise: [Yes/No]

Reflection:

....

....

....

....

....

....

Day 30: Challenges and Adjustments

Date: [Enter Date]

Mood: [Enter Mood]

Difficulties Encountered:

- Struggles with maintaining the regimen: [Yes/No]
- Any adverse reactions or side effects: [Yes/No]

Adjustments Made:

- Changes to the remedy dosage or preparation: [Yes/No]
- Modifications to diet or exercise routine: [Yes/No]

Positive Changes Noted:

- Significant improvements in symptoms: [Yes/No]
- Positive feedback from others: [Yes/No]

Reflection:

....

....

....

....

....